Tips to Save Your Life

in Times of Danger

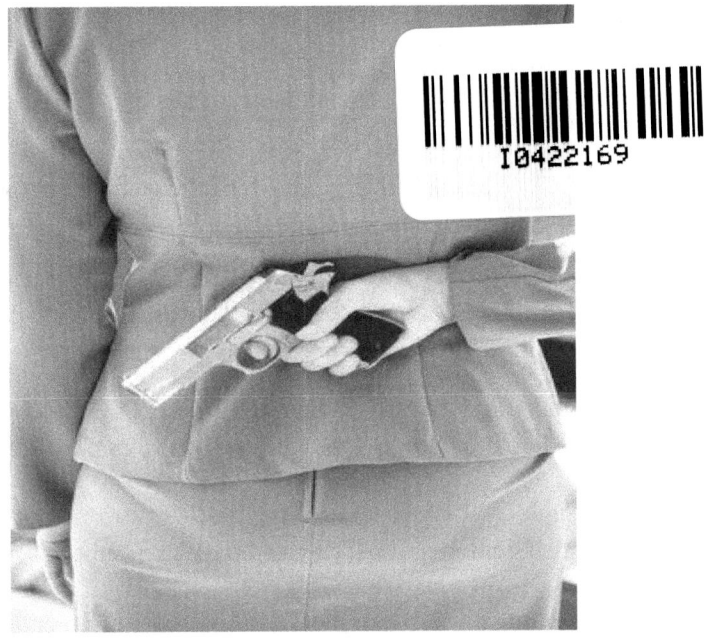

Prepping and Survival Series

M. Usman

Mendon Cottage Books

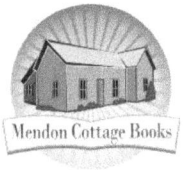

JD-Biz Publishing

Disclaimer

The information is this book is provided for informational purposes only. It is not intended to be used and medical advice or a substitute for proper medical treatment by a qualified health care provider. The information is believed to be accurate as presented based on research by the author.

The contents have not been evaluated by the U.S. Food and Drug Administration or any other Government or Health Organization and the contents in this book are not to be used to treat cure or prevent disease.

The author or publisher is not responsible for the use or safety of any diet, procedure or treatment mentioned in this book. The author or publisher is not responsible for errors or omissions that may exist.

Warning

The Book is for informational purposes only and before taking on any diet, treatment or medical procedure, it is recommended to consult with your primary health care provider.

Our books are available at

1. Amazon.com
2. Barnes and Noble
3. Itunes
4. Kobo
5. Smashwords
6. Google Play Books

Table of Contents

Preface...4

Tips to Save a Life 5

    Chapter # 1: Water 5

    Chapter # 2: Fire..9

    Chapter # 3: Cold 13

    Chapter # 4: Earthquake...16

    Chapter # 5: Surviving Hot Temperatures 19

    Chapter #6: Surviving a War..22

    Chapter # 7: Defeating the Jungle..25

    Chapter # 8: Surviving a Car Accident 28

Preparation 30

    Chapter # 9: How to Pack an Emergency Kit 30

Conclusion 33

Author Bio...34

Publisher..45

Preface

If you have ever survived a life and death situation, then you know how shocking the moment can be. It always feels like the type of thing you only see on TV, until it starts happening. You might try forcing yourself to think that you are watching a horror movie, only to realize that it is happening in your face. As it happens, there is one thing that stays in the back of the mind – how is this going to end?

While there are others who have cheated death and told stories of moments like these, not everyone is so lucky. But, putting luck aside, knowing just how to act during the moment might be all you need to get out of such tragic situations alive. These might include road accidents, fires, floods, etc.

There is no guarantee that the information in this book will save you. However, it is a fact that everything presented might increase your chances of survival. In this book, you will learn tips you can apply in different life-threatening situations. At the end, we will look at how you can prepare for disasters.

So, read on.

Tips to Save a Life

Chapter # 1: Water

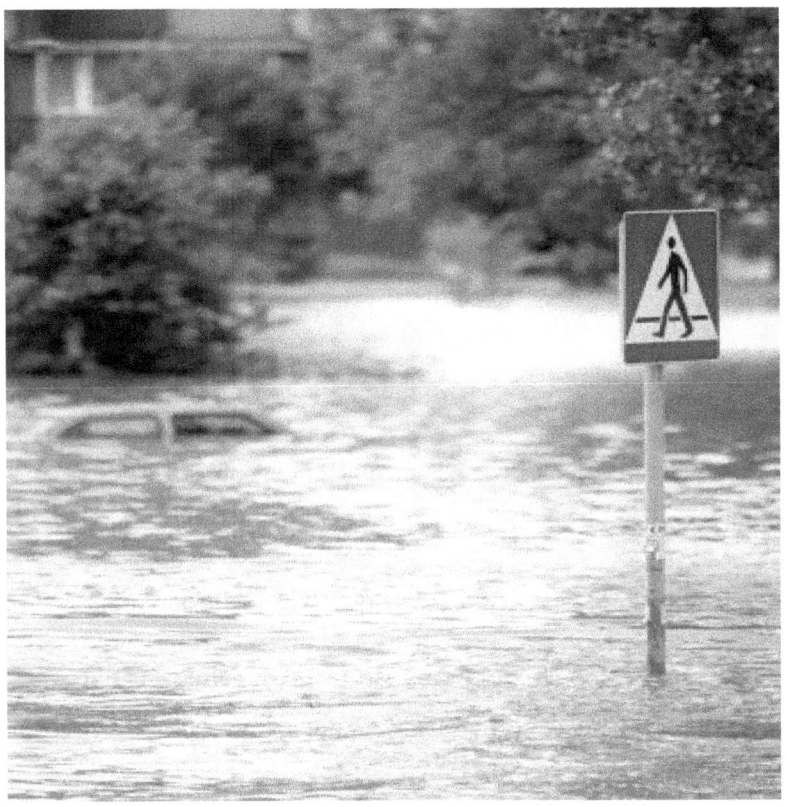

There are a million ways to die and water related deaths are among the top ranking killers. Water accounts for an estimated 372,000 deaths annually. Based on statistics, it is the third leading cause of unintentional injury death all over the world.

What makes water even scarier is that we are surrounded by it all the time. So, it helps to have a few tricks up your sleeve to pull out in times you find yourself in a life or death situation with this beast.

Water can kill in many ways. However, drowning is the most common form where water claims the majority of its victims. This usually happens when people go swimming or during accidents while traveling on water. But in some situations, it brings the danger to us in the form of floods - destroying property and lives in the process.

Flooding is very dangerous and has the ability to turn an entire neighborhood into a graveyard, in a matter of hours. However, with a little know-how, you can survive any water attack.

Swimming

Year after year, we hear stories of family vacations ending tragically, as a result of drowning in seas, oceans, or lakes. In most situations, however, these deaths are avoidable. The problem is that people neglect the basics and forget that the same water that keeps us alive can turn deadly in an instant.

Here are some tips to follow if you want to swim again another day:

- ***Alcohol and Swimming Don't Interact***: It is true that opposites work well together - but that does not apply when it comes to swimming while drunk. Apparently, most of the drowning deaths occur because someone tried to do it while drunk. Alcohol reduces your ability to react or to change effectively, thereby increasing the chances of an accident. So, if you want to drink, resist the urge to get in the water. If you cannot, then..

- ***Never Swim Alone***: It does not matter if you have been swimming for thousands of years – things can go wrong in the water. As a matter of fact, there are a number of veteran swimmers who have died as a result of drowning. So, as a precaution, take someone with you when going into the water. This is also true for kids.

- ***Breathe***: In the event that the worst has happened and you are drowning, try to breathe. This works in two ways: you will not panic so you will respond better to the situation and it will keep you buoyant, reducing your chances of drowning.

- ***Lay on Your Back***: This helps you breathe.

- ***Don't Raise Your Hands***: If in a standing position, never try to raise your hands up - that will increase the chances of drowning. Rather, spread them out and keep them flat in the water. This will also keep your head above the water. If you can, swim to safety. Use your feet as well, since your hands will tire easily, leaving you vulnerable.

Flooding

Flooding incidences have been increasing in recent years. Unlike drowning in the sea, these do not only take away lives, but infrastructure and personal property as well. As if that is not enough, floods usually claim a lot of lives. However, it is still possible to survive a flood in some situations. Here are some things to keep in mind:

- ***Follow the Weather Forecast***: Despite the fact that nobody knows how the weather will turn out, the National Weather Service is usually on track with its predictions. So if they say a flood is about to happen, take it serious. This is very true if you live in a low-lying area. If you can, move to a higher land.

- ***Never Walk in Moving Water***: During the flood, it is never a good idea to walk in moving water, even when it is going slowly. If such water can carry vehicles away, it is even worse for humans.

- ***Use a Stick When Walking***: Find a long stick and use it to detect how firm the ground is before stepping on it. Floods are known to wash roads and bridges away making drowning very easy.

- ***Stay Away From Electric Equipment***: Water is a good conductor of electricity, so unnecessarily touching electric equipment will be all it takes to pull the life out of you. This also applies to power lines. If you need to turn an appliance off, use the main switch.

- ***Look out for Animals***: Flooding usually brings a whole jungle of animals into residential areas. In most cases, it is snakes that find their way into people's homes, so be extra careful wherever you go.

Chapter # 2: Fire

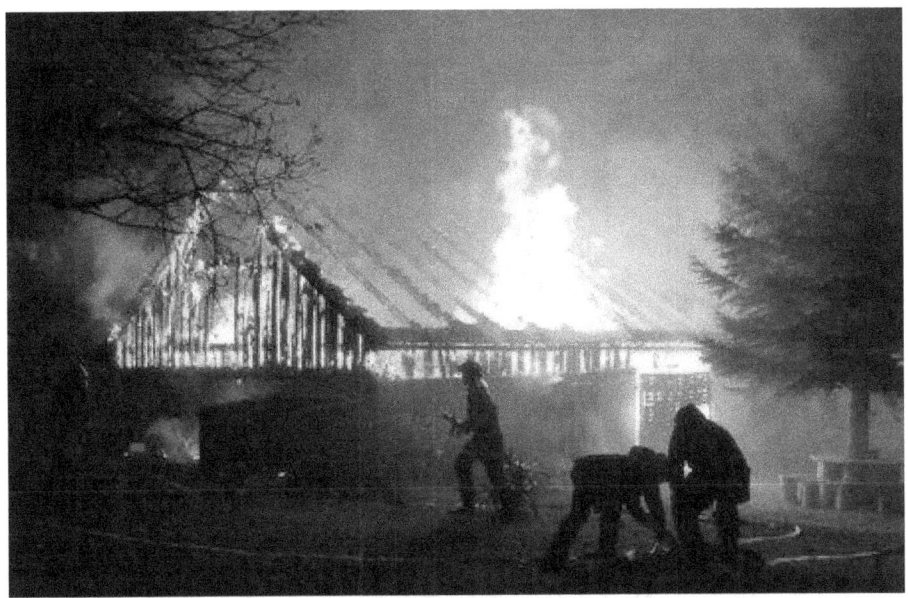

It can be said that no amount of planning is guaranteed to save you, but as we all know, knowledge is power, and its presence or lack of it, might change your chances of survival. Each year, lives are lost as a result of fires.

Contrary to popular belief, the majority of deaths in a fire are not a result of burns. Rather, it is the heavy smoke that takes away people's lives. Simply inhaling the heavy smoke a couple of times is enough to leave you unconscious. When that happens, the actual fire is what comes next, as there is no other way of escaping it.

With some preparation and a few tips, you can take a gamble and walk out of a fire in one piece.

Preparation

Unlike with car accidents, which usually occur on the road or boat accidents which only sink in water, fires do not discriminate. They will come to life almost anywhere, which is why they are very dangerous. To make it even worse, they start when you least expect it.

But as with everything, preparation is the best key to defeating them. This chapter will focus on house fires, as they are the most common and deadliest.

Here are some things to consider, even if you believe your house cannot catch fire:

- *Install Smoke Alarms*: Having smoke detectors is one of the easiest things you can have in order to know when a fire starts. Inspect them from time to time to make sure they still work.

- *Know The Escape Routes*: Since it is your house, you must already know how to get out in times of danger. If you have visitors, let them know the fastest way to escape the house in case a fire starts.

- *Keep All Keys Close*: While locking doors is a good way to stay safe from outside dangers, you should realize that you can be trapped when the danger is inside. So make sure everyone knows where you keep the keys. Preferably, leave them on the doors.

- *Have Fire Extinguishers*: This can never be over emphasized. If you cannot have one in each room, then simply get as many as you can.

- *Keep Doors Closed*: While it is counterproductive in that you will not know in case fire starts in another room, closing doors slows its progress.

- *Practice Fire Drills*: This is especially true if you have kids or elderly in the house. And as a bonus, it is kind of fun doing it with the whole family

During the Fire

All the above mentioned was to help you in case you have a fire in your house. However, the way you act during the moment is just as important. Below are some tips you have to follow:

- *Stay Low*: If you never missed any science classes, then you might know that hot air rises, leaving cold air at the bottom. In this case, the hot air is the smoke, so stay as low as you can when getting out of a burning house.

- *Cover Mouth and Nose*: Apparently, it is not enough to simply stay low, so soak a cloth in water and use it to cover your nose and mouth. This will block the inhalation of harmful smokes.

- *STOP, DROP, ROLL*: If your clothes catch fire, remember to do these three things; stop, drop and roll. That will help put the fire out. Hide your face with the hands as you do this.

- *Stay Away From the Elevator*: You should never try to use the elevator in an effort to escape a fire. Instead, go for the stairs if they are free from fire and smoke.

- *Be careful When Opening Doors*: When trying to open a door, use the back of your hand to feel how hot it is. If it is hot, stay away from it. But even when it is not, open it slowly and be ready to close it in case fire and smoke rushes in.

- *Keep Smoke Out With Wet Towels*: If trapped in a room, use wet towels or clothes to close any openings. These are the spaces that could facilitate the entry of smoke.

- ***Have Water Handy***: If you do not have a fire extinguisher in the room, then keep some water in a bucket or bathtub, if there is one. Use this to put out any fire in the room.

- ***Jump Out From the Window***: While it is not recommended to jump from anything above the second floor, sometimes you may have no choice. If you think you can make it, give it a shot. First, make sure there are no obstructions in your way and before taking the plunge, hang from the window first, and then jump.

- ***Signal from The Window***: If you cannot jump, then use a flashlight, cloth, or shout to get attention from those who can save you.

Chapter # 3: Cold

Despite the fact that cold weather can be lovely sometimes, it can also be deadly in some situations. As a matter of fact, people have died as a result of it. The good thing is that these cases are rare, because almost everyone knows how dangerous cold weather can be. When it happens, most of the time it is because the victims had no other choice of keeping themselves warm.

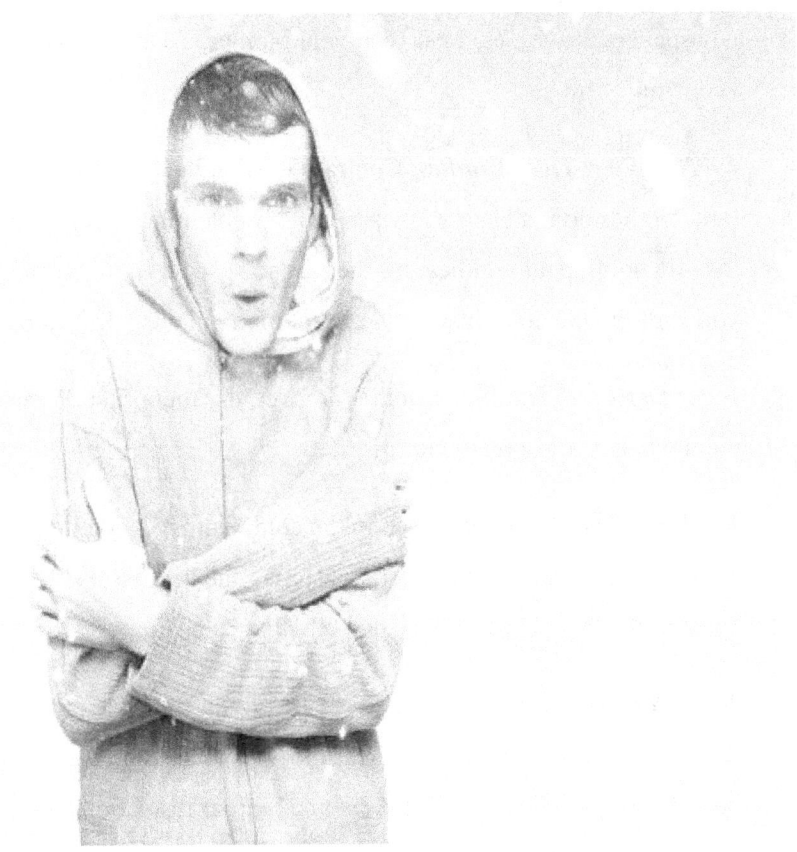

This chapter will focus on how you can protect yourself from the cold when stuck outside. So without further ado, here are the tips:

- **Build a Shelter**: It does not need to be pretty- forget about looks and focus on functionality. The material you will use depends on where you are. If you can find cardboard, go with it, but if that is not an option, then use whatever is available. This could be sticks, leaves, plastic bags, grass, etc. And to ensure that it keeps heat, make it very small.

- **_Wear as Many Clothes as You Can_**: This is an old trick that works every time, but since nobody goes out with a whole suitcase of clothes, you might need to improvise. You can try stuffing newspapers, leaves, etc., between your clothes. That should help keep you warm.

- **_Do Not Wear Tight Clothes_**: Contrary to what you would think, tight clothes do not keep you warm. The problem lies in the fact that they do not trap a lot of heat, as there is no space left. In the end, you start feeling cold. Instead, go for clothing that is a little loose.

- **_Wear Dry Clothes_**: If your clothes are wet, dry them first. Wearing them when wet is a recipe for disaster.

- **_Keep the Head Covered_**: When in the cold, almost everyone focuses on the legs, hands and the chest, neglecting the head. But shockingly, that is one part of the body that is losing heat.

- **_Never Sleep on the Ground_**: Use whatever you can find, but try not to sleep on a bare floor. So, find cardboard, clothes, or even make a bed of leaves. The trick is to have some kind of insulation between you and the ground.

- **_Stay Hydrated_**: Many like to think that because it is cold drinking water is not necessary, but this is wrong. You need water just as you do when it is hot.

- *Fire*: It is probably the best remedy man has invented for cold weather. But, since you might not always have a match handy to start a fire, learn to do it in the old way in advance – using sticks and stones.

Chapter # 4: Earthquake

Of all the natural disasters, earthquakes are among the most difficult to predict. An earthquake hits when you least expect it. Although it normally lasts only a few seconds or minutes, an earthquake is still capable of taking an unimaginable number of lives, in that short time. Just like floods, earthquakes destroy buildings and other people's property as well.

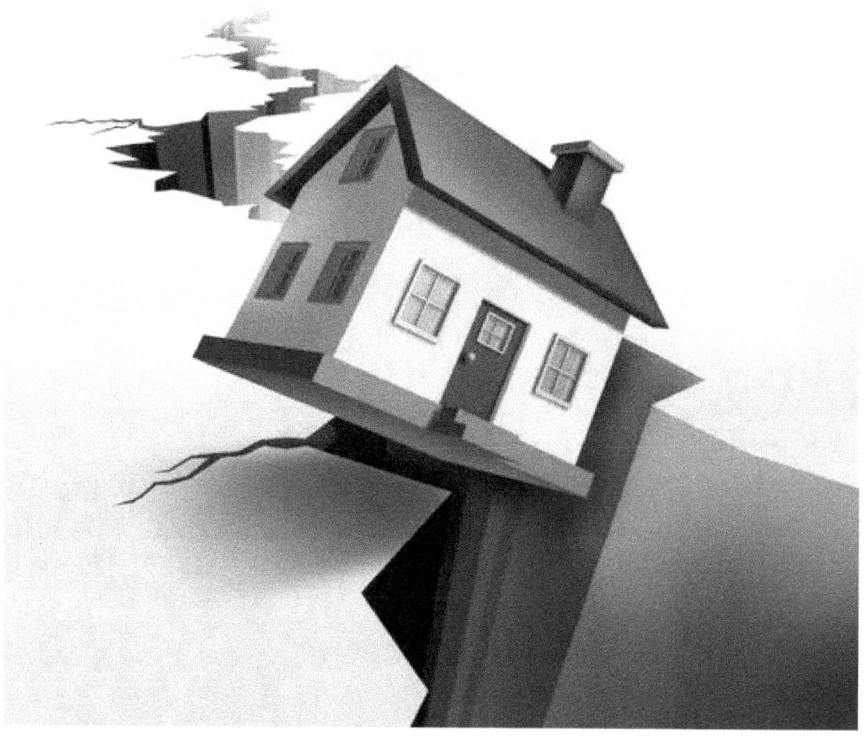

While it takes luck to survive an earthquake most of the time, having a little how-to info could be all you need to make it out alive when it occurs. Usually, a quake will find you inside a building or when you are outdoors. The chances of surviving in each of these situations will depend on its magnitude and your surroundings.

Outside

If you are outdoors, you have a much higher chance of surviving, as long as you are free from things that could crash into you. Here are a few tips to keep in mind:

- *Get to an Open Space*: Your first priority should be to get to an open area. Look around and assess whether there is a chance of buildings, trees, power lines, or other things falling on you.

- *Avoid Moving Around When in a Safe Place*: Once you are somewhere believed to be safe, avoid moving around. You could easily fall and get injured because of the violent shaking of the ground.

- *Avoiding Hiding Under Bridges*: Since some bridges are earthquake proof, many believe hiding under these is the way to go. But in some situations, these could be just as vulnerable, so stay away.

- *Stay in the Car*: If you are in a car when it happens, simply move it to a safe spot and stop driving. It's safer being in there than standing outside. Just make sure you are not blocking the road.

- *Get Away From Coastlines*: Depending on the earthquake, there is a chance of a tsunami if you are at the beach. So try to get to safer land as soon as you can, until it is declared safe to go back.

Indoors

Buildings are probably the worst affected when an earthquake occurs. So, if you are inside, simply do not panic. It is possible to get out of a falling building alive. Here is what you should do:

- ***Drop, Cover, and Hold***: This is the recommended way of surviving a quake if you are inside a building. Simply get down under a solid structure (table, bed, desk, or other forms of furniture) and stay there. Remember to cover your head and neck and hold on to the thing you are hiding under.

- ***Do Not Try to Run Outside***: While there is always the temptation to run outside in the thick of things, you should resist that urge. You will likely fall and expose yourself to danger.

- ***Avoid Electric Equipment***: There is a chance that electric appliances and cords will be broken in the process, so avoid touching these, as you could easily get electrocuted.

- ***Prepare for the Aftershock***: Almost all big earthquakes will have an aftershock. These aftershocks can bring down a house after the main quake is long gone. So stay alert.

- ***Avoid Walls***: When trying to get out, stay away from the walls. They could already be destroyed just waiting for a simple push to come down.

Chapter # 5: Surviving Hot Temperatures

It is a fact that the majority of land around the world is turning into deserts, and with current trends, this will likely get worse. Unfortunately as humans, we cannot cope with the high temperatures associated with these areas. That is the reason many die when lost in deserts.

It is rare for anyone to die in his or her home as a result of hot temperatures. This is partly because we have air conditioners, water, and shelter, which are crucial in the survival of high temperatures.

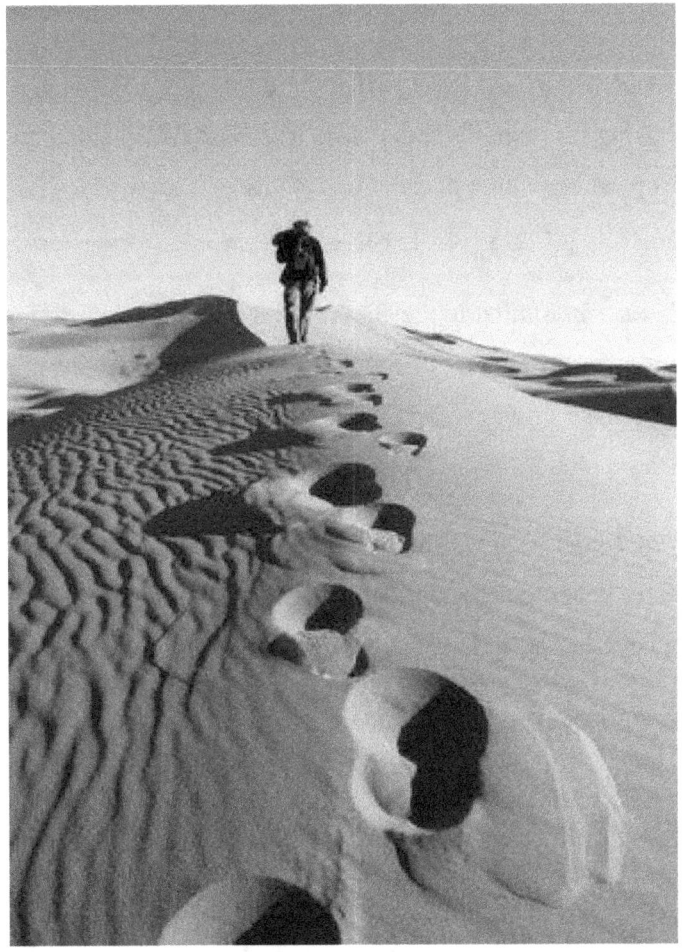

But in the desert, there are no such luxuries.

You might find yourself stuck in this no man's land as a result of a car break down, plane crash, etc. So what does a person do when all around is sand, little or no trees, and water is scarce?

Here are the things to do when stuck in a desert:

- *Stay Hydrated*: Since hot temperatures will make you lose a lot of water quickly, you should try to stay hydrated all the time. But, remember that finding water in a desert is not that easy, so use what you have sparingly. You are better off without food than water.

- *Avoid Strenuous Activity*: If you are walking, go slowly. If you are looking for food, it's better to do it at night when temperatures have dropped. Any high demanding activity will leave you with less water, reducing your chances of survival.

- *Cover Up*: Similar to the above, cover up your head and body. That will limit the amount of water you will lose through evaporation. But, make sure your clothing is loose and bright colored to reflect heat.

- *Stay Under a Shed*: Similar to the above, find a shed and hide under it. It's better to come out in the evening when it is a bit cooler. If you have a car, use it.

- *Keep Warm During The Night*: Ironically, the desert is one of the coldest places during the night, so be prepared for this as the sun goes down.

- *Look Out For Animals*: From snakes to scorpions and everything in between, make sure you are ready for it all. For your information, these animals have learned the art of survival – they come out in the night when temperatures are bearable.

- **Signal for Help**: Knowing how to let people see you from afar is a good way to make it out alive. So find a mirror, CD, or any chrome-coated plate, and use it. It will create a bright light that will let those far away see you and know that you need help. Additionally, you can start a fire.

- **Make your Way Traceable**: If you decide to move in search of civilization, mark you way in case somebody comes to find you. You can place stones at every given interval, for example. Additionally, it will help if you decide to come back.

- **Don't Just Drink any Water**: If you are thinking of drinking desert water, remember that it might be contaminated. So if you do it, be aware of the consequences. As a precaution, start a fire and boil it first.

- **Keep Mouth Shut**: You will lose a lot of water through your mouth, so if possible, keep it shut at all times.

Chapter #6: Surviving a War

The world is no longer a safe place. Just watch the news and you will realize how violent man has become. You just do not know when a nuclear bomb might go off in your neighborhood. Adding to that, not everyone gets years of training in the military on how he or she can survive a war, thus leaving average people with no option but wait for their fate.

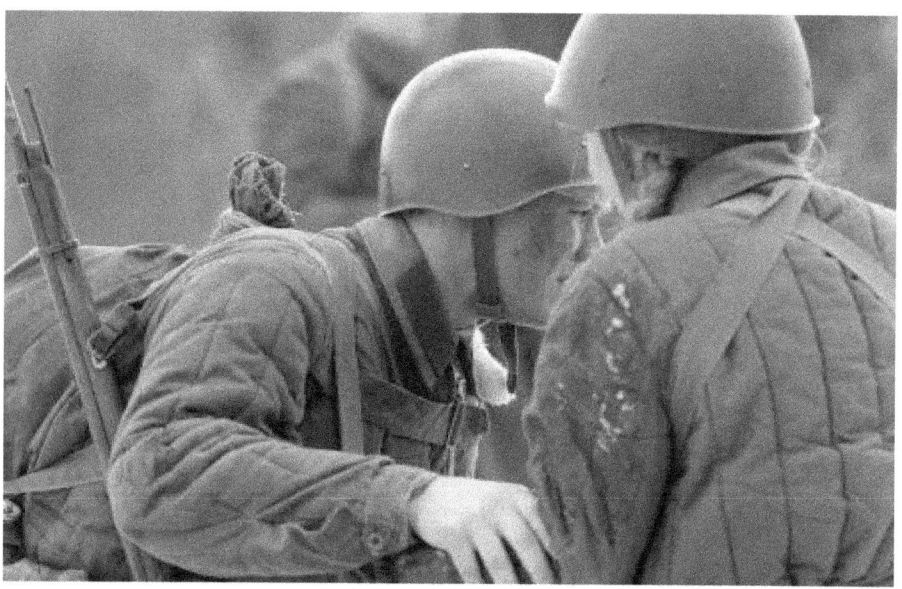

Having a few tricks in your repertoire can get you out of a war zone, so you tell about it another day. Here are some tips for surviving a war:

- **_Do Not Panic_**: If you have ever been caught in the line of fire, then you know how tense the moment can be. It is easy to lose your mind and act subconsciously in this kind of a situation. Seeing somebody's blood flowing is enough to freak you out and start you running aimlessly all over the place. Unfortunately, this is the best way to get killed, so try to breathe and make sense of the situation.

- **_Find Cover_**: Your first bet should be to find some cover near you.

Usually, a wall is enough if the guns being used are not that powerful. And as a precaution, stay low at all times.

- *Get Away*: Whoever is shooting at you might eventually get where you are, so try to get away as soon as you think it is safe. It is recommended that you crawl on your belly as you do this.

- *Hit The Ground*: If there isn't a wall or something you can use as a shield, it is best to get on the ground as soon as possible. Do not think of running when someone is shooting at you or you will get shot. Rather, get away by crawling on your belly. And if there are explosions involved in the equation, the ground is your only best friend.

- *Hide*: If you cannot run away, the best thing to do is hide. Desperate times call for desperate measures – for example, hide under dead bodies. Each situation will be different so think outside the box.

- *Stay hydrated*: Since you will be moving a lot, it is crucial to drink water at all times.

- *Eat What You Have*: You will likely lose a lot of energy in a war, so if possible, eat whatever you find, even when you are not feeling hungry.

- *Go Somewhere Safe*: If you have a chance, it is best to run where you believe you will be safe. It is the only guaranteed way of surviving a war.

- *Watch the News*: To avoid surprises, make it a point to stay informed with what is happening around you. You will know when a war is imminent.

Chapter # 7: Defeating the Jungle

Life can take a twist when you least expect it. You would never imagine yourself stuck deep in the Amazon forest or some other dense jungle around the world. However, that is possible. We have seen planes crashing in these places, leaving passengers to survive on their own. If this was to happen to you, the only thing to protect you from the dangers of the forest is your survival skills.

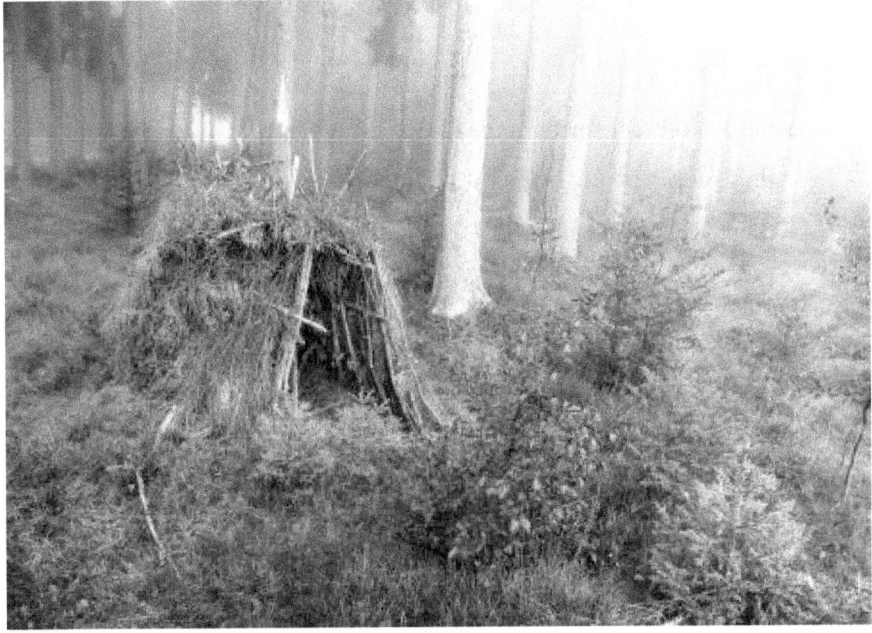

Therefore, it does not hurt to know just enough to get you out of that kind of a situation. So without further ado, let's get started:

- **Have a Weapon**: There are lots of dangerous animals in the jungle. If you have a gun, very well - it is among the best defense weapons man ever made. But if you do not, there is another option. Find a long stick and shape its tip into a spear. Make sure it is strong enough to take any kind of punishment. You will need this even if you have a gun.

- ***Hydration is Key***: Studies have shown that man can live for weeks without food, but he will only last days without water. So do whatever you can to find some water if you already do not have it. You can let a plant condense it for you or get it from a river. Just make sure you boil it to kill bacteria.

- ***Start a Fire***: Boiling water means you should know how to start a fire. Not only that, but it will also keep you warm when it is cold.

- ***Find Food***: Just as with water, finding food in the jungle is not that hard. You will find a range of plants and fruits. However, some of these could be poisonous so stick to what you know. Additionally, there are a lot of animals you can eat. If you still want more, find a river and try fishing by making a pronged fishing spear.

- ***Build a Shelter***: It is not a good idea to keep walking at night in the jungle. So if you can, find a good place to build a shelter. Just make sure there is no risk of trees or branches falling on you.

- ***Keep Clothes On***: No matter how hot it gets, never try to remove your clothes. There are spiders, snakes, mosquitoes, and so many other dangers, waiting to get a piece of you.

- ***Follow A Reference Point***: If you have ever heard stories of people getting lost in the jungle, then you must also have heard about how difficult it is to avoid walking in circles. Not only does this make you lose the little energy you have, but also it is demotivating. So before you even start your journey, identify a reference point in the distance and follow it.

- ***Use a Stick When Walking***: Do not use your hands or any part of the body in making your way through the thick dense of the forest. Rather, use a stick, as you just do not know what may be hiding there.

- ***Do Not Make Noise***: If a tree falls in the forest and nobody is there to hear it, does it make a sound? So if you know there is no one around, do not bother making noise. You will only put yourself at the mercy of animals that will track you.

- ***Do Not Rush***: It is understandable that you might want to get out as soon as possible. But, do not rush as you might fall and get injured in the process.

- ***Cross Rivers Carefully***: Use your stick to determine how deep a river is. If in doubt, figure out another way. The risks are many and include drowning, an attack by territorial hippos, but most importantly, crocodiles.

Chapter # 8: Surviving a Car Accident

Without question, road accidents take away just as many lives as diseases. This is no surprise, considering that we depend on cars as the most convenient form of transportation.

Sadly, every time we get in a car, we increase our chances of an accident. We might try as much as we want to avoid one, but we should remember that there are drunks using the same road, poor conditional vehicles, and many other factors, all facilitating the occurrence of an accident.

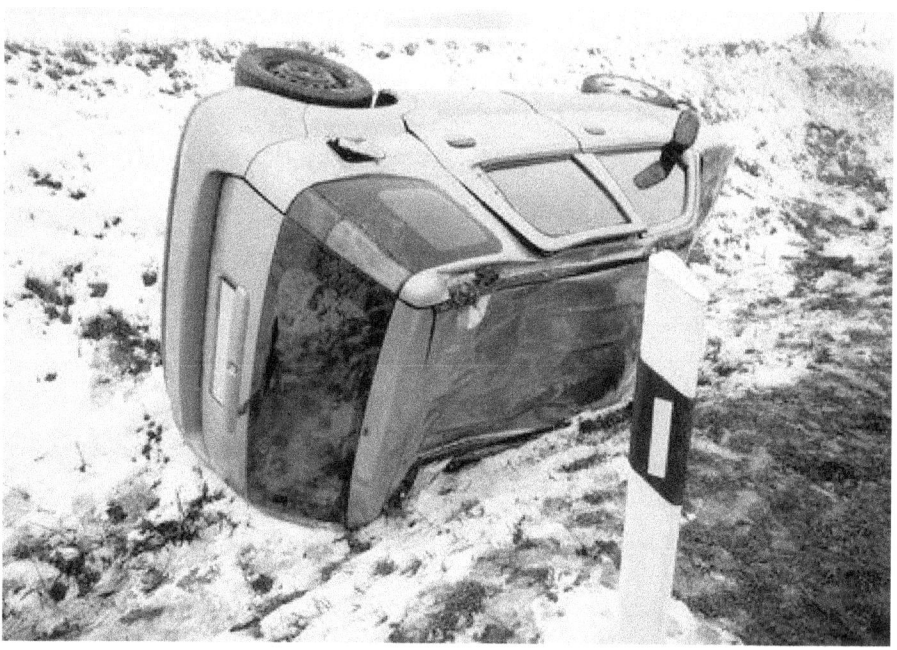

But as with everything, preparation and avoiding panic are the only ways to survive such tragic events: So, here are the tips:

- ***Wear Seat Belt***: Accidents happen quickly, leaving you with little or no time to respond effectively. Wearing a seatbelt is the best way to ensure that you stay in your seat as it happens. And as a driver, encourage your passengers to do the same.

- *Seat Properly*: Simply wearing a seatbelt is not enough. For it to work effectively, you should be sitting upright – not leaning forward, backward, or to the side. Additionally, not sitting properly means you will get in the way of an airbag when it comes out.

- *Be Careful with Missiles*: Any free object in your car could become a missile and injure you during an accident. To avoid such an occurrence, keep these kinds of objects in the trunk or behind seats.

- *Avoid Head-on Collisions*: Usually, you will know when an accident is imminent. So if possible, try to avoid a head-on collision. But, at the same time, do not position the car so it ends in a sideways collision - that will even be worse as cars are structurally weak on the sides.

- *Control Speed*: Forces of nature dictate the faster something goes, the more kinetic energy it has, so if involved in an accident, the damage will be significant. Therefore, simply reducing your speed will increase your chances of survival.

- *Maintain your Car Regularly*: Not all accidents are a result of the drivers being at fault. Some can be traced to the car not being in a good condition.

- *Never Drink and Drive*: It has been said a countless number of times, but still, people drink and drive. If you know you will be drinking, have someone sober drive you.

Preparation

Chapter # 9: How to Pack an Emergency Kit

As seen in this book, we are subject to dangers that may hit us in the blink of an eye. It is, therefore, crucial that we spend more time planning, so that when disaster strikes, we will have more time escaping. One thing you should always prepare in advance is an emergency kit.

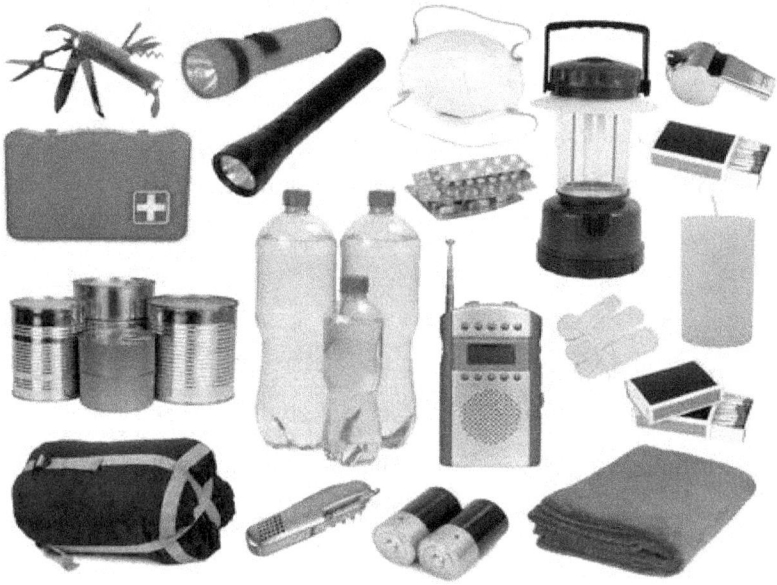

Building an emergency kit that covers every situation is difficult. So, your efforts should focus on making one that will get you through the type of disaster likely to hit you. If your area has a history of floods, think of what you will need if they happen again. If prone to earthquakes, then you will have to include things to cover that as well. I am sure you get the idea.

Your emergency kit is supposed to last at least 72 hours. To get you started, here are some things you should include:

- *Water*: As evident in this book, hydration is important. The recommendation is that a single person should use one gallon of water per day for drinking and sanitation. The more people there are, the more water you will need to pack.

- **Food**: It should be nonperishable and remember to change it at least once a year.

- *First Aid Kit*: There may be no time to take every injury to the hospital during a disaster, and hospitals are usually overwhelmed when a lot of people have been affected. So, have a first aid kit that includes gloves, bandages, medication, etc.

- *Local Maps*: They will come handy when trying to figure out your way.

- *Whistle*: Not absolutely necessary, but may prove important when trying to communicate. And hey, it does not take much space.

- *Pliers and Wrench*: These are always needed for a range of tools.

- *Flashlight*: Even if you run out of space, do what you can to find a place for this and remember to include extra batteries.

- *Battery Powered Radio*: A disaster does not mean you should be completely separated from the rest of the world. Additionally, you will need to know how things are progressing.

- *Sleeping Bag*: Include one for each member of your house and be sure the bags are suitable for outdoor use.

- *Knife*: You will use this for making a shelter and more.

- *Important Phone Numbers*: This could be the phone numbers of those who, you believe, will have the capacity to help you.

- **_Emergency Reference Book_**: It is not as if you will always know how to do everything. So pack this as well for quick reference.

With everything included, your emergency kit should still be portable and accessible by anyone. If you know there is something you might not live without, be sure to include it in the kit.

Conclusion

The tips in this book are some you can use to stay safe in times of danger. As stated at the beginning, there is no guarantee that the information in this book will ensure survival. Rather, it only increases your chances of making it out in one piece. Of all the tips, however, you should always prepare in advance. Danger is always knocking on our door and there is no one who can be exact of when it will happen. Make sure you watch the news all the time, as floods, wars, and other types of disasters can be seen coming.

Author Bio

Muhammad Usman is a distinguished medical graduate of Allama Iqbal medical college (AIMC). He is a professional writer who has been in the field for more than 4 years. During this time he has produced 10,000+ articles, blogs and eBooks on various niches related to diseases, health, fitness, nutrition and well-being. He is a regular contributor to several journals related to medicine and surgery. He is the editor of several journals and newspapers.

Check out some of the other JD-Biz Publishing books

Gardening Series on Amazon

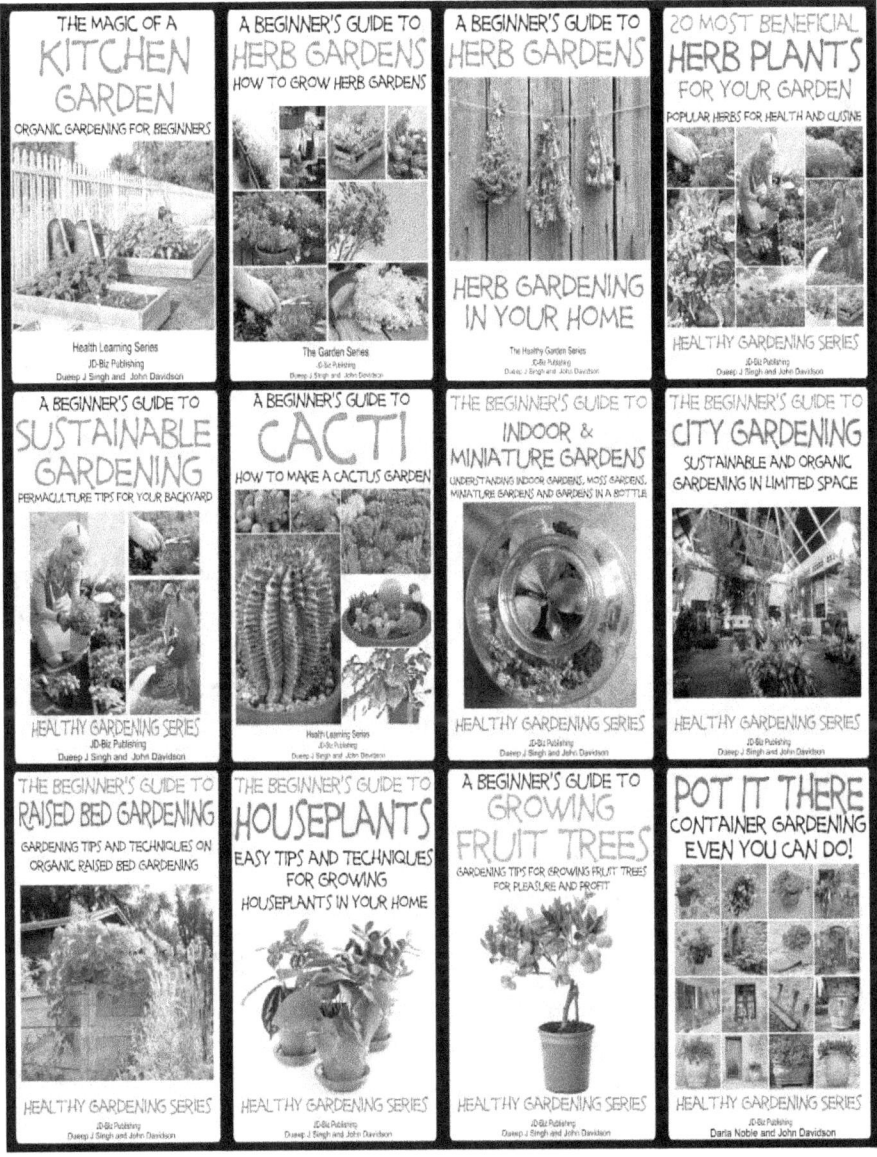

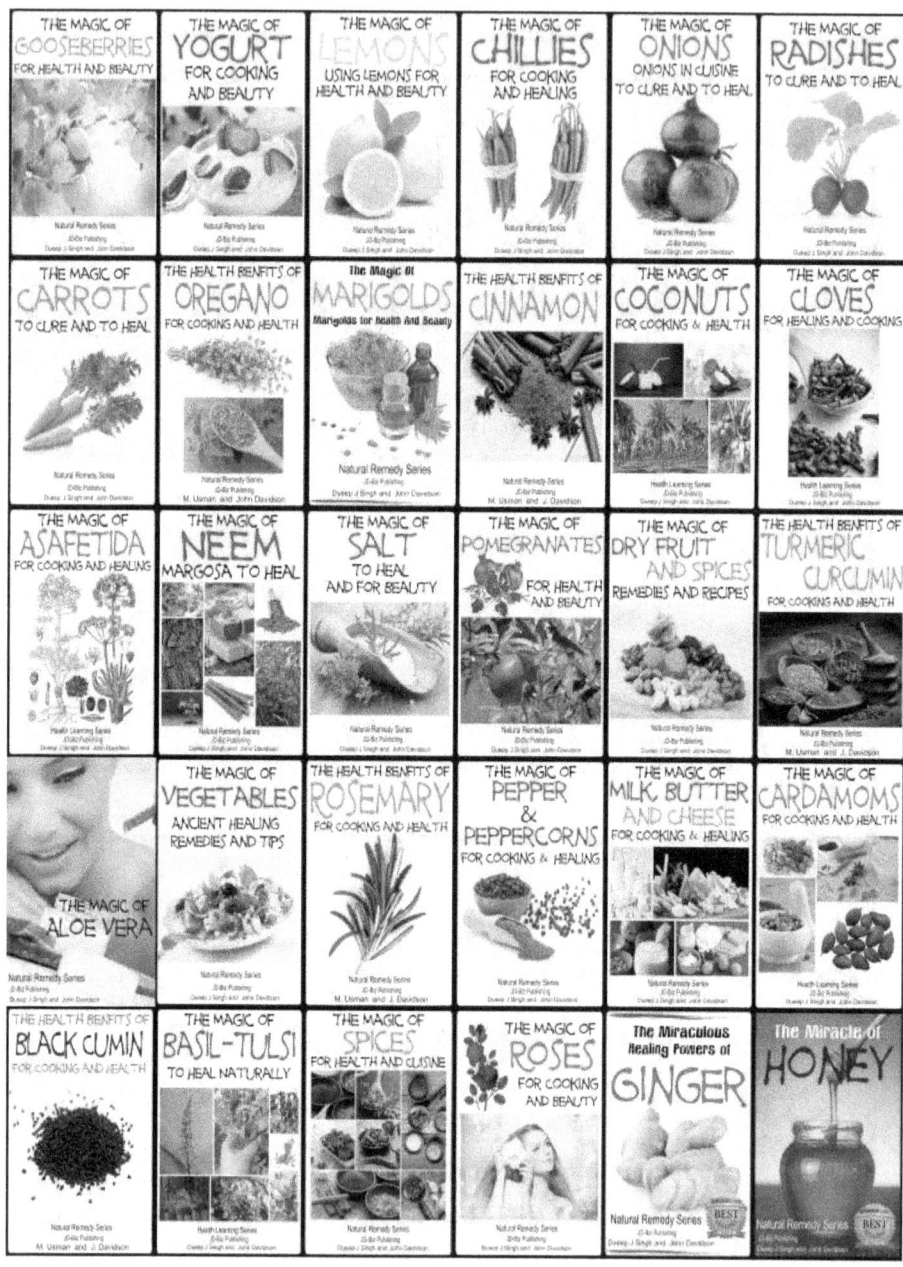

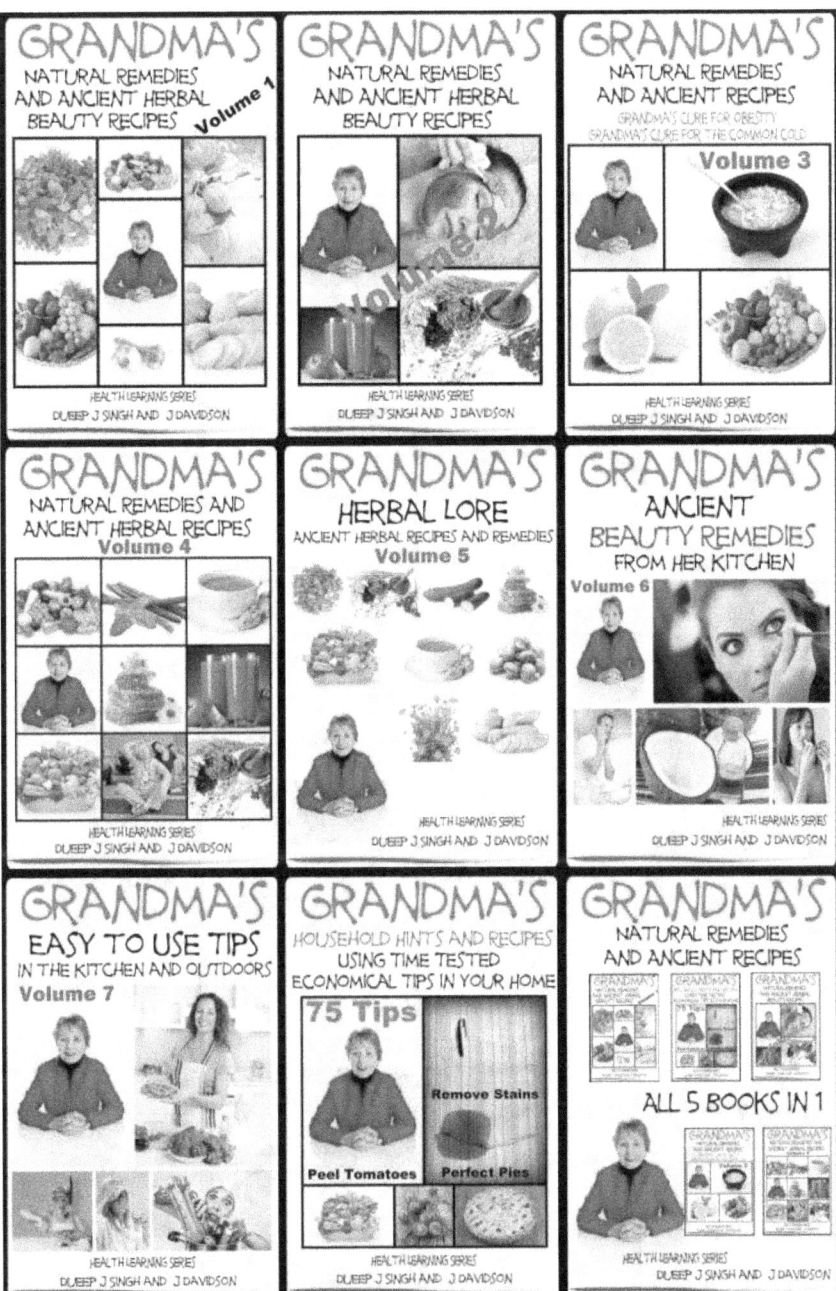

Country Life Books

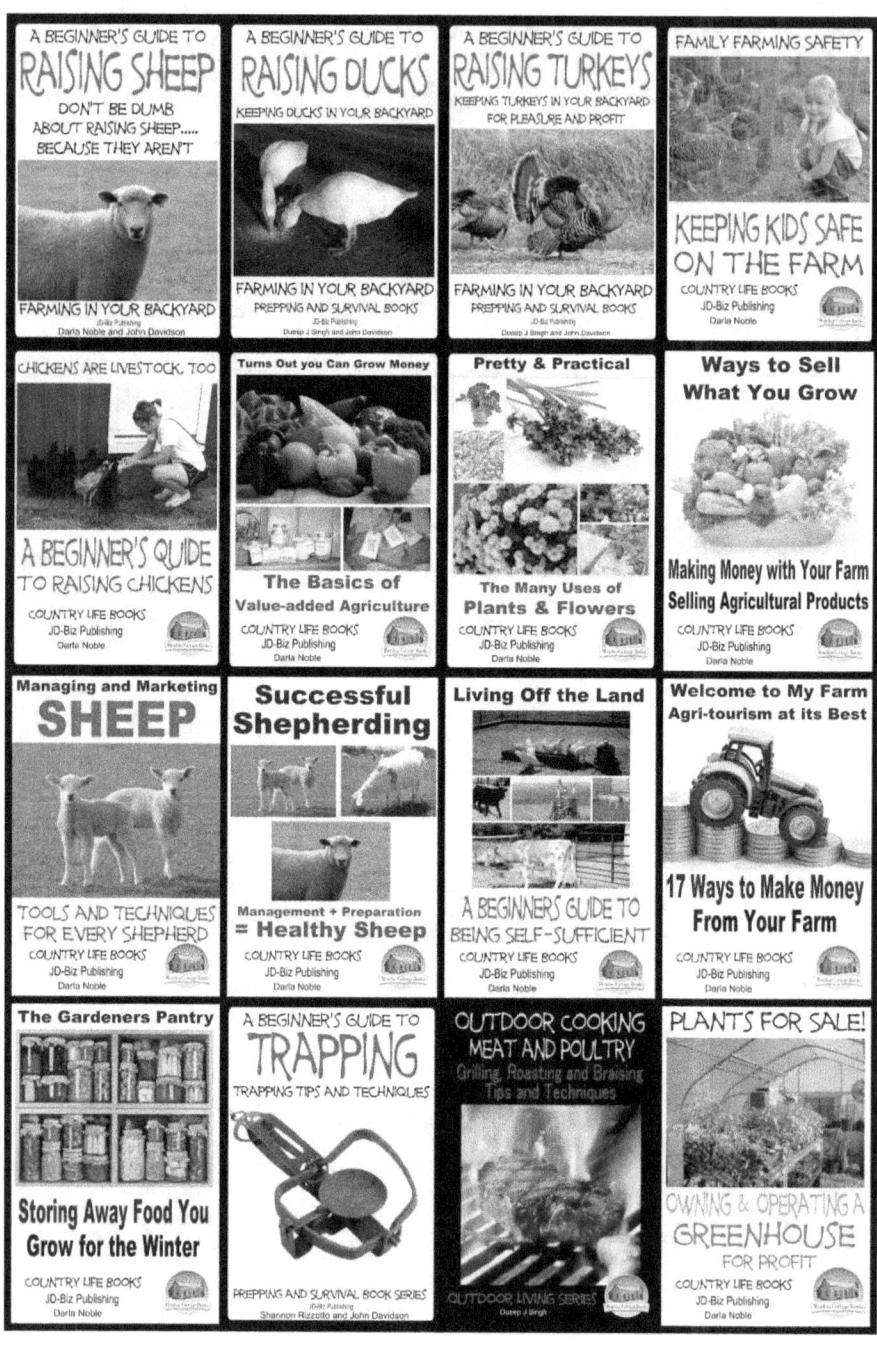

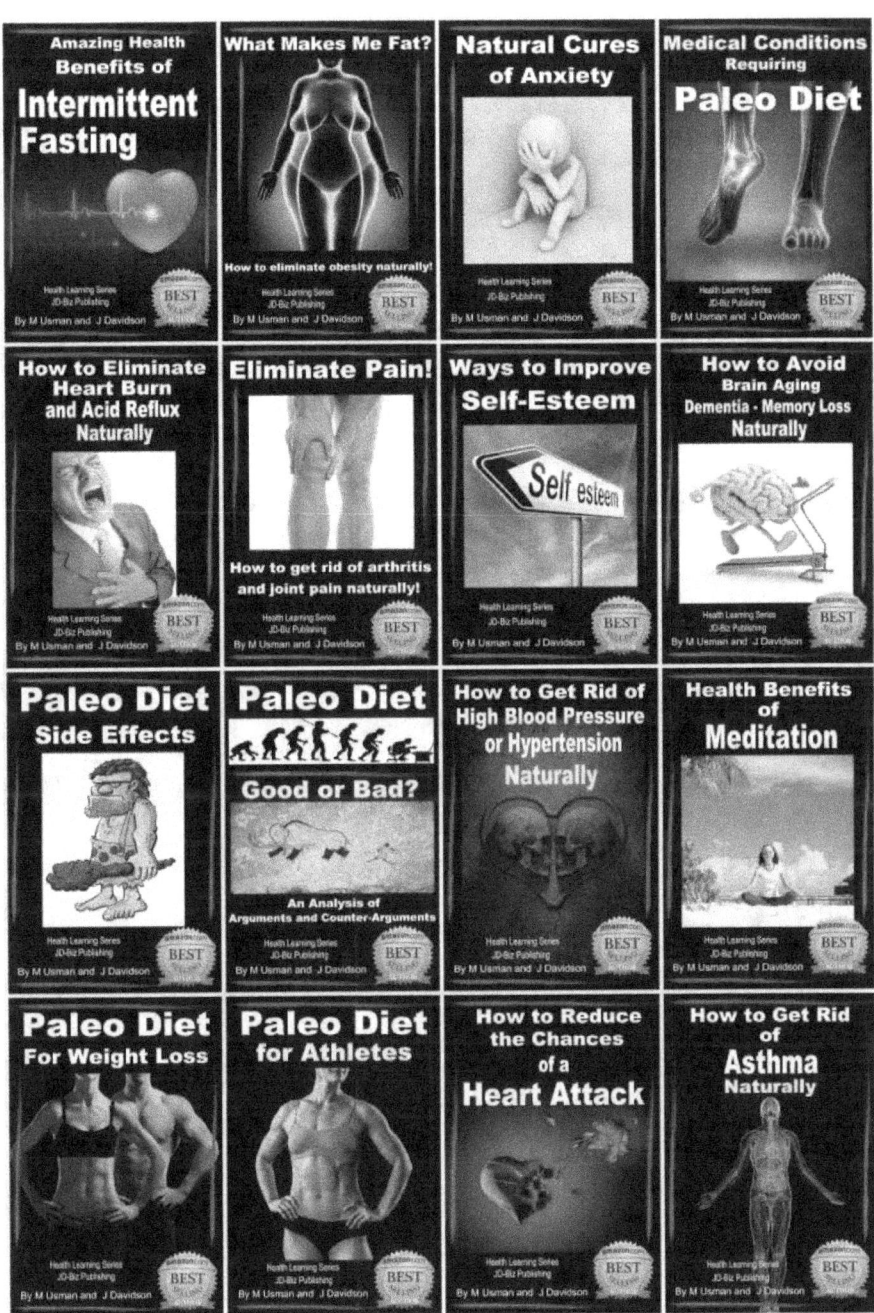

Amazing Animal Book Series

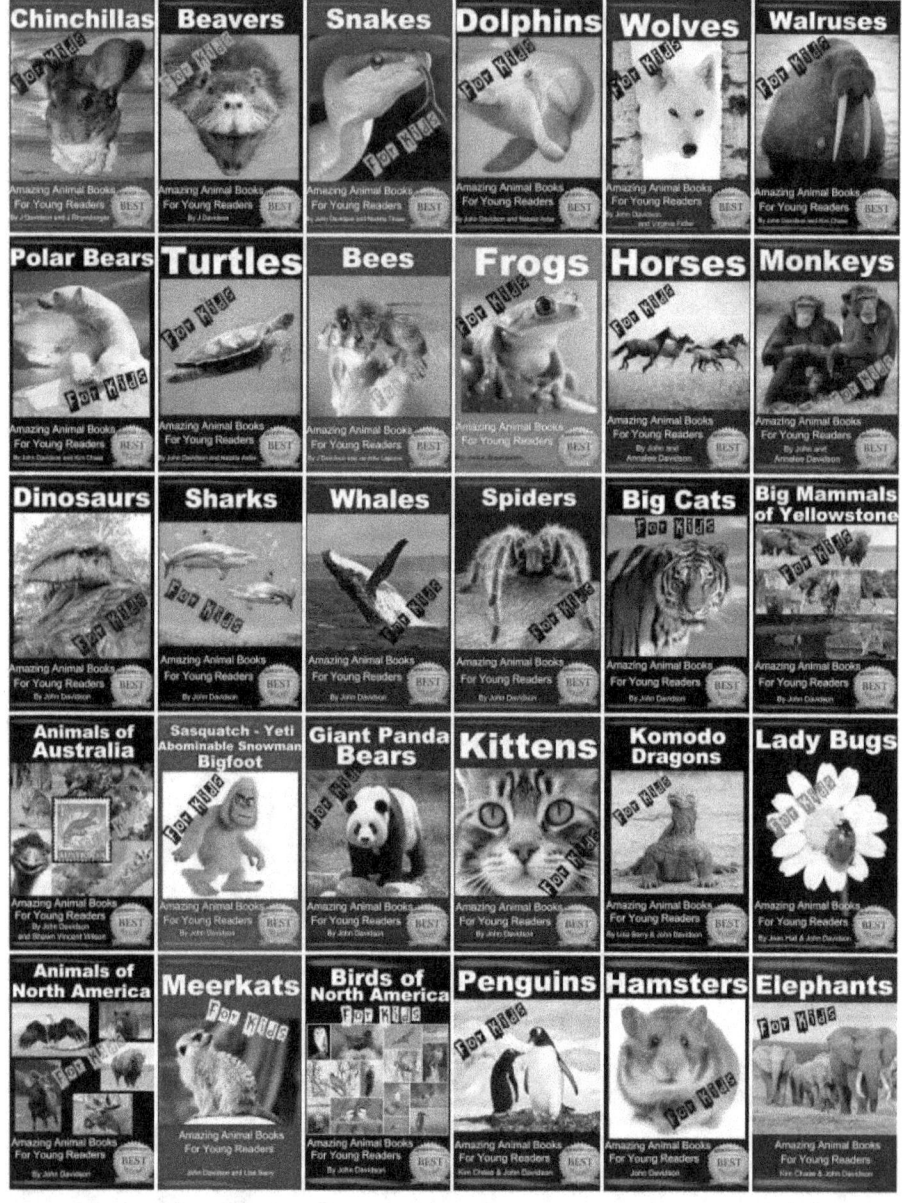

Learn To Draw Series

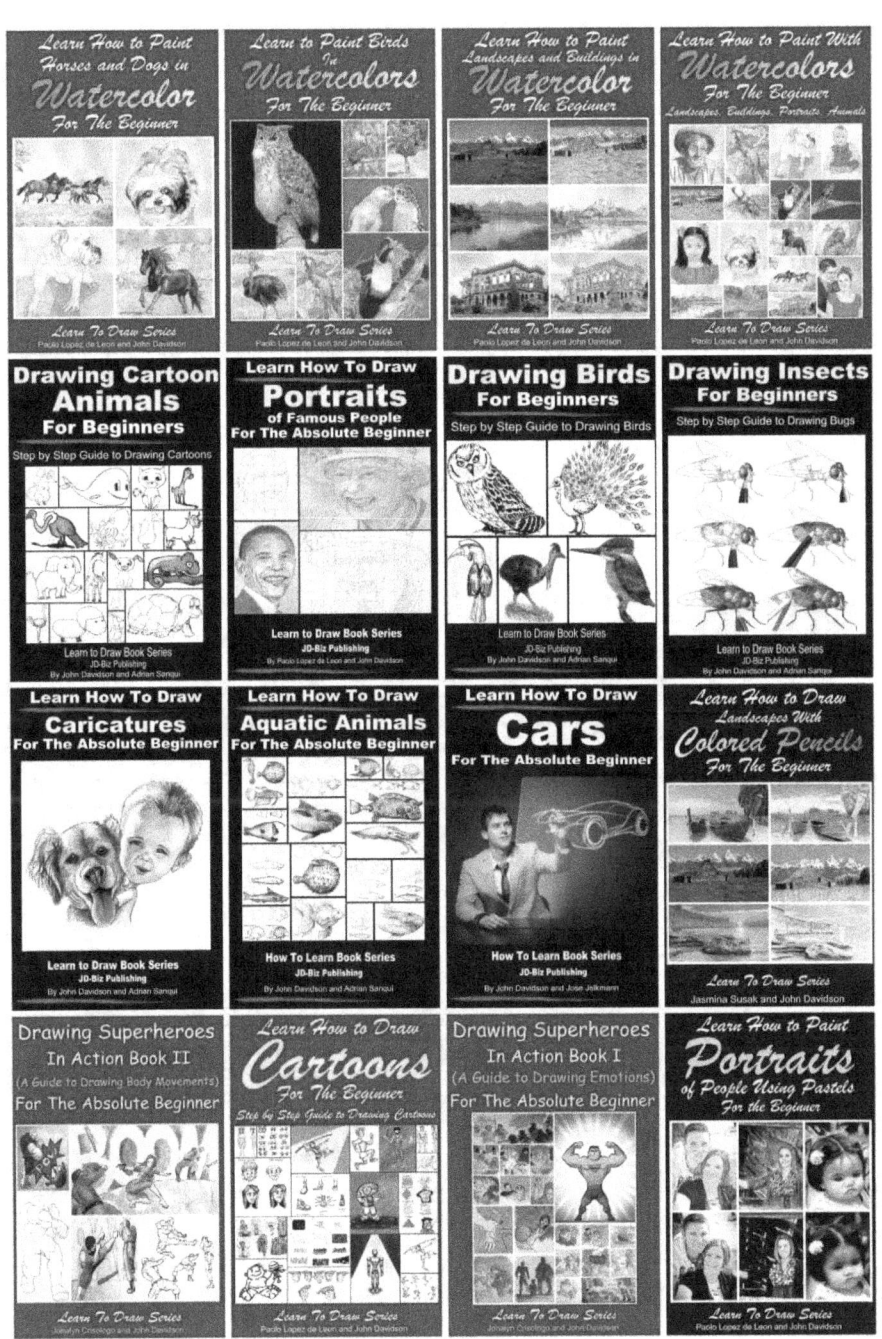

How to Build and Plan Books

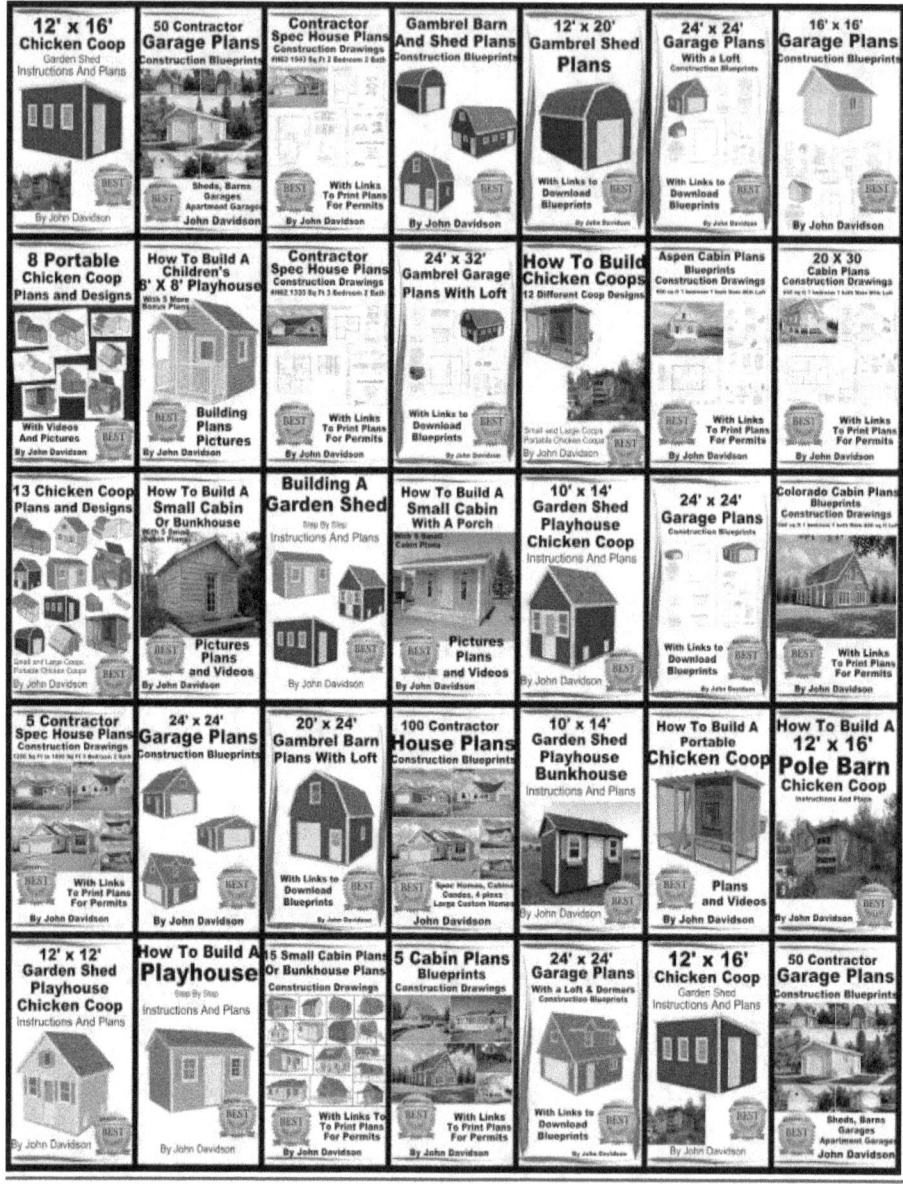

Entrepreneur Book Series

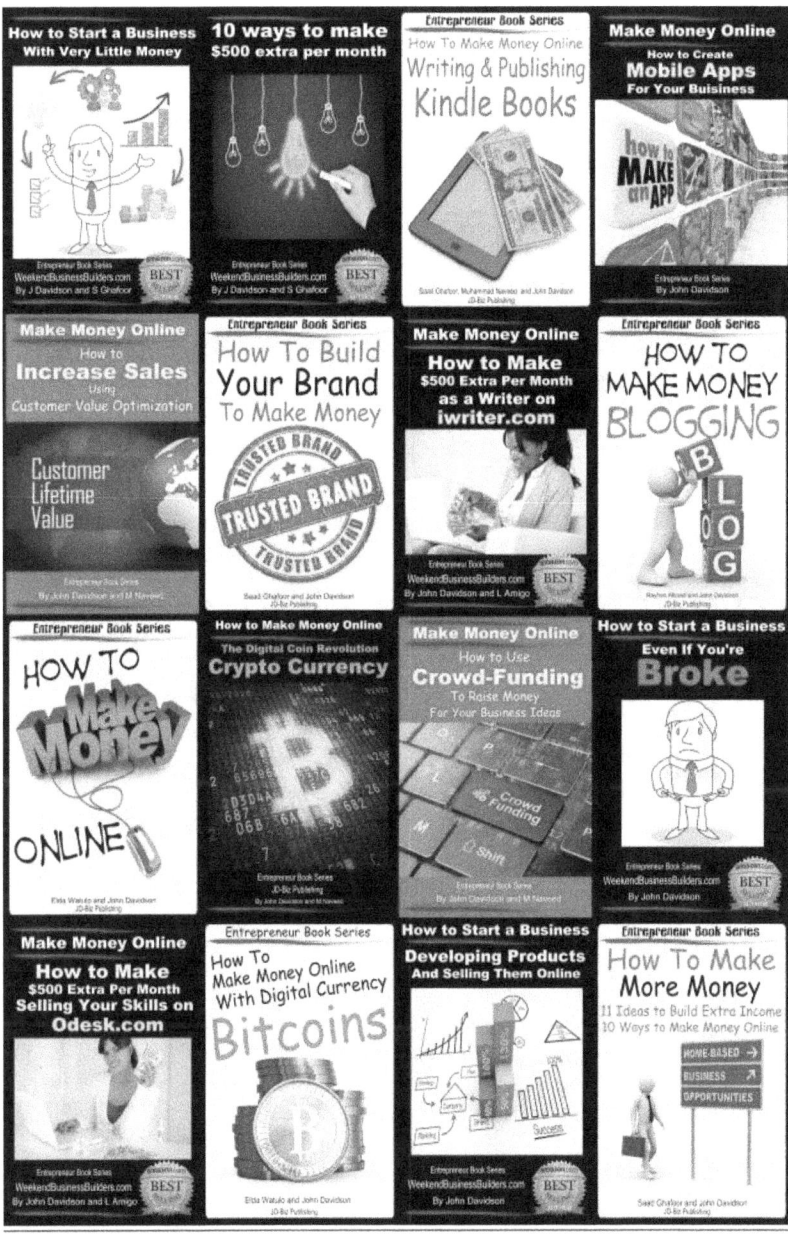

Our books are available at

1. Amazon.com

2. Barnes and Noble

3. Itunes

4. Kobo

5. Smashwords

6. Google Play Books

Publisher

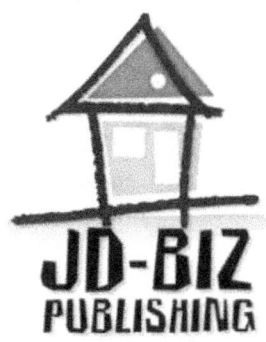

JD-Biz Corp

P O Box 374

Mendon, Utah 84325

http://www.jd-biz.com/

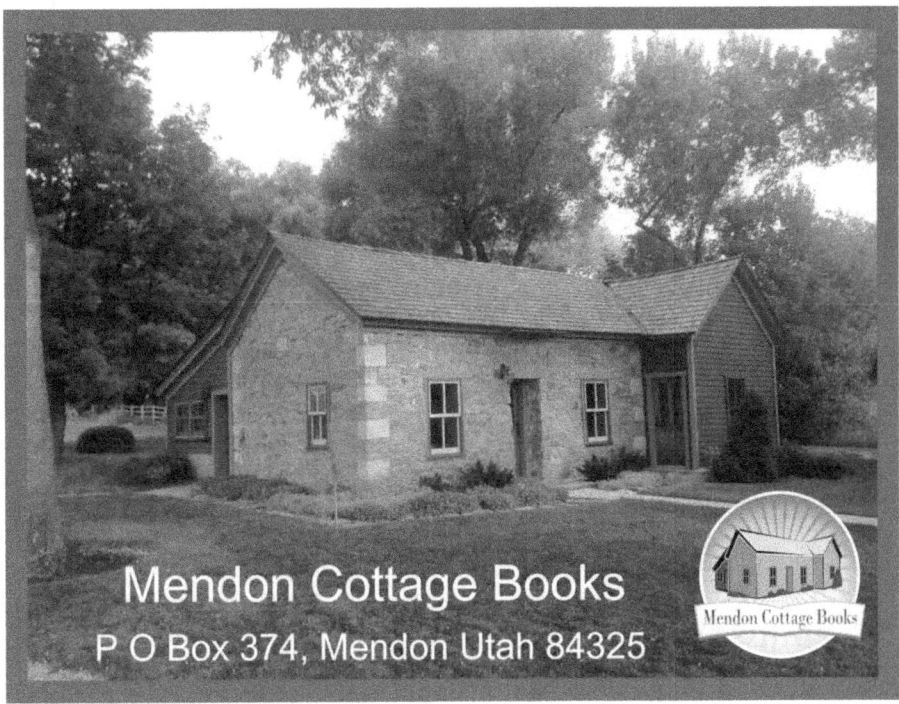

Mendon Cottage Books

P O Box 374, Mendon Utah 84325